Father,

Thank you for 
strength and wisdom we gain from training.

*Be with us as we work that we may do our best.
Help us to be encouraging to others in our daily
life. Thank you for the people that you have
brought into our lives.*

*Bless the athletes, coaches, workout partners
and all those who support our training.
May the results from our training be a
reflection of Your Spirit in our lives.*

*Finally Father, remind us that there is no
failure, but only growth in the body, mind and
Spirit.*

Amen

Copyright

Tactical Cross Training WOD Bible: Hardcore Workouts for Spartan Warriors, Action Heroes & Special Forces

Second Edition – September 2014.

Written by P Selter

Disclaimer

The information provided in this book is designed to provide helpful information on the subjects discussed. This book is not meant to be used, nor should it be used, to diagnose or treat any medical condition. For diagnosis or treatment of any medical problem, consult your own physician. The publisher and author are not responsible for any specific health or allergy needs that may require medical supervision and are not liable for any damages or negative consequences from any treatment, action, application or preparation, to any person reading or following the information in this book. References are provided for informational purposes only and do not constitute endorsement of any websites or other sources. Readers should be aware that the websites listed in this book may change.

I recommend consulting a doctor to assess and/or identify any health related issues prior to making any dramatic changes to your diet or exercise regime.

Contents

Your Free Gift

As a way of saying thanks for your purchase, I'm offering a free report that's exclusive to my readers.

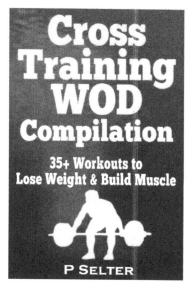

You can download this free report by going here.

www.WODBible.com

Fitness gurus always want to make out that getting in shape and working out is harder than it really is, **that's why I wrote:**

Cross Training WOD Compilation: 35+ Workouts to Lose Weight & Build Muscle

This book is a handy little reference containing the workouts and info to get started on your journey today; I encourage you to share this bonus report with your friends & family too!

As this is a limited time offer it would be a shame to miss out, I recommend grabbing this bonus before reading on.

PS: I'm always adding additional workouts and tips to my books, by clicking on the link above I'll also be able to send you an updated version of the eBook you've purchased free of charge.

Introduction

I would like to thank you and congratulate you for purchasing the book, **Tactical Cross Training WOD Bible.**

This book will introduce you to the many health & fitness benefits of the phenomenon that is Cross Training, along with 150 Tactical Cross Training WODs (workouts) you can implement immediately to improve your speed, strength and agility.

These workouts are designed to improve your functional strength, power & agility.

Many workouts out there are designed for the vanity of the mirror, they're designed to make you look good, yet leave you with all 'show' and no 'go' when it comes to athletics and functional strength.

You'll not only develop an unbreakable body via these workouts, but also a determined mind that'll help you push through any endeavor or adversity you face in your life.

Thanks again for purchasing this book, I hope you enjoy it!

Benefits of Cross Training

Cross Training is not just a new fad amongst all the other styles of training that come and go throughout the years; Cross Training has many benefits these include:

Intensity

Cross Training workouts are fast paced and intense (as the emphasis is on speed and total weight being lifted), they are generally much shorter than a regular weight lifting workout – however since the workout is condensed it is constant non-stop movement, there is no time to stop and talk to your gym partner between sets like you normally would as you are constantly working against the clock to better yourself.

Creates Athletes

Cross Training exercises are all high power functional movements, this is highly emphasised. Cross Training, unlike bodybuilding does not believe in low power isolation movements. The major benefit here is now that the focus has been taken off vanity and looks it has been put 100% on performance – the core strength, stamina, coordination, agility and balance you will develop through participation in Cross Training will transfer over to sports and all other facets of life.

Time

The number one excuse for individuals not following a workout regime is the constraint of time; yes its true – working out takes time. However, Cross Training WODs are short - with many intense workouts ranging from 15 – 20 minutes they are faster and more effective than a regular workout in which you spend an hour on a cross trainer mindlessly staring at the wall.

Measureable Results

Cross Training workouts provide you with measureable and repeatable data; this can be used to verify that your fitness level is increasing. With a series of 'bench mark' workouts known as 'The Girls' and 'The Heroes' you can easily assess your progress.

Life Changing

Change your body, change your life, and change your world...
Cross Training workouts build mental strength, grit and confidence; a tough Cross Training workout will emotionally push you beyond your limits. When you ignore the voice inside your head that says 'it's too hard' or 'I can't do that last rep' and push past it unbreakable confidence is built – then anything is possible.

Community

Cross Training encourages community, both in the gym and online. People encourage and support each other through out their workouts – you will never have to work out alone again unless you want to, as the bond formed between training partners make training truly fun. It is very rarely you will find an individual that is as passionate about a particular pastime as yourself however this could not be further from the truth with the Cross Training community; we are all teammates that push and pray for each other.

The Importance of Tactical Training

Tactical training is exactly as it sounds – if you want a tactical edge in your sport, military career, martial arts or just everyday life performing functional movements in both explosive power style workouts along with extended endurance style training is paramount.

You won't find any useless biceps curls or triceps extensions in these tactical workouts, we're here to build strength, power and endurance to get us out of the line of military fire, we're here to ensure our body is forged strong enough to prevent the opposing team from scoring that goal at the last second.

The enemy whom comes unprepared will always falter to you so long as you put in the hard yard and focus on the tactical workouts on offer in this book.

Second place is no longer an option.

Terminology

The following Cross Training terminology guide will come in helpful when interpreting your Tactical Cross Training workouts.

1RM: Your 1RM is your max lift for one rep

AHAP: as heavy as possible

AMRAP: As many rounds as possible

ATG: Ass to Grass

BP: Bench press

Box: Another name for a gym

BS: Back squat

BW: Body weight

CTT: Cross Training Total - consisting of max squat, press, and deadlift

CTWU: Cross Training Warm-up

Chipper: A WOD containing many different exercises and reps

CLN: Clean

C&J: Clean and jerk

C2: Concept II rowing machine

DL: Deadlift

DOMS: Delayed onset muscle soreness

DU: Double under

EMOM: Every minute on the minute

For Time: Timed workout, perform as quickly as possible and record score.

FS: Front squat

GHR(D): Glute ham raise (developer). Posterior chain exercise, similar to a back extension. Also, the device that allows for the proper performance of a Glute Ham Raise.

GHR(D) Situp: Situp performed on the GHR(D) bench.

GPP: General physical preparedness, another word for fitness

GTG: Grease the Groove, a protocol of doing many sub-maximal sets of an exercise throughout the day

H2H: Hand to hand; refers to Jeff Martone's kettlebell "juggling" techniques

HSPU: Hand stand push up. Kick up into a handstand (use wall for balance, if needed) bend arms until nose touches floor and push back up.

HSQ: Hang squat (clean or snatch). Start with bar "at the hang," about knee height. Initiate pull. As the bar rises drop into a full squat and catch the bar in the racked position. From there, rise to a standing position

IF: Intermittent Fasting

KB: Kettlebell

KBS: Kettlebell swing

KTE: Knees to elbows.

MetCon: Metabolic Conditioning workout

MP: Military press

MU: Muscle ups. Hanging from rings you do a combination pull-up and dip so you end in an upright support.

OH: Overhead

OHS: Overhead squat. Full-depth squat performed while arms are locked out in a wide grip press position above (and usually behind) the head.

PC: Power clean

Pd: Pood, weight measure for kettlebells

PR: Personal record

PP: Push press

PSN: Power snatch

PU: Pull-ups or push ups depending on the context in WOD

Rep: Repetition. One performance of an exercise.

RM: Repetition maximum.

ROM: Range of motion.

Rx'd: As prescribed, without any adjustments.

SDHP: Sumo deadlift high pull

Set: A number of repetitions. e.g., 34sets of 8 reps, often seen as 4x8, means you do 8 reps, rest, repeat, rest, repeat, rest, repeat.

SPP: Specific physical preparedness, aka skill training.

SN: Snatch

SQ: Squat

SS: Starting Strength; Mark Rippetoe's great book on strength training basics

Subbed: Substituted

T2B: Toes to bar. Hang from bar. Bending only at waist raise your toes to touch the bar, slowly lower them and repeat.

Tabata: A form of interval training comprised of 20 seconds on, 10 seconds off repeated for 8 rounds.

TGU: Turkish get-up

The Girls: A series of benchmark workouts named after girls

The Heroes: Brutal benchmark workouts in honour of fallen soldiers

TnG: Touch and go, no pausing between reps

WO: Workout

WOD: Workout of the day

YBF: You'll Be Fine

Scalability

On the following pages you will find 150 Tactical WODs.

All of these workouts are entirely scalable, if you're unable to reach the specified repetition range, distance, use the weight listed or find yourself unable to continue for the duration of rounds/time listed I recommend scaling the workout to suit your current fitness level.

The movements included in each and every one of these workouts are functional – if necessary alter the weight and any other factors you deem necessary, however keep the core exercises the same.

That said do not be lazy and reduce the workload of the WODs for no reason.

None of these workouts are easy, they are not designed to be easy... they're designed to give you the strength, power and agility you need to dominant life.

Pay the price today in your workouts and enjoy the fruits of your labor tomorrow when you're kicking ass.

If a regular workout is a light cup of coffee that slowly wakes you up, Cross Training is a shot of five-hour energy!

Tactical WODs

WOD 1

Rope Climb X25ft

Step Ups X15ea

Sandbag Clean X10-15

Hanging Leg Raise X15-20

400M Run

Repeat 7-10 times

If you do not have a rope you can sub with pull ups and sandbag clean with barbell or KB cleans

WOD 2

Deadlift> 4-5X8-12

 Pull Ups> 4-5XSubMax Mixed Grip

Jump Squat X 15

Inverted Rows X SubMax Mixed Grip

 Push Press X 20

Walking Lunges JX15ea

Bear Crawl X100 ft

15 Mins AMRAP

WOD 3

Sandbag Squat> 4-5X15

Sandbag Overhead Press> 4-5X10-15

 Burpee> 4-5X5

Step Ups> 4-5X15ex

Single Arm Bent Over DB/KB Row> 4-5X8-12ea

Burpee> 4-5X5

2 Mile Ruck Run

WOD 4

KB Swing X10-15

High Pull X10 ea arm

Clean X10 ea arm

Snatch X10 ea

Press X10 ea

Overhead Carry X100ft

 Burpees X5

25 mins AMRAP

WOD 5

KB Clean 2 Squat X15

Pull Ups/ Muslce Ups XSubMax

Box Jumps X15

Decline Push Ups XSubMax

Wall Walks XSubMax

200M Sprint

35 mins As Many Rounds As Possible (AMRAP)

WOD 6

Sandbag/Barbell Overhead Strict Press 4X5-8

Overhead Pull Aparts 4X25

Hanging Leg Raise 4X15

Pull Ups 4XSubMax

Pull Aparts 2.0 4X10-15

Burpees 5X10

DB Shrugs 5X12-15

Run The Rack DB Curls 3X8-8-8-8

WOD 7

Sandbag Shoulder Squat 5X10 each

Hanging Leg Raise 5X15-20

Alternating Reverse Lunge 5X15/15

Banded/Chain Push Ups 5XSubMax

Med Ball Slams/Sledge Hammer 5X20

Single Arm Overhead Carry 5X50ft each

Burpees 5X10

WOD 8

Push Ups X100

Walking Lunges X50ea

Pull Ups X50

Jump Squat X50

Burpees X60

Flutter Kicks X100

Complete as fast as possible

WOD 9

Sandbag Clean & Press X100 (Women:30lbs Men:60lbs)

Sandbag Carry X10min (Women:30lbs Men:60lbs)

Break down 1 and 2 in any way, complete for time.

 Run 1600M

Push Ups X100

Pull Ups X50

Break down 1-3 in any way, complete for time

WOD 10

Bench> 4X5-8

Bent Over 1 Arm DB Row> 4X12-15ea

Incline DB Bench> 4-5X15

BB Row Wide Overhand> 4-5X12-15

Decline Sit Ups> 4-5X15

Dips> 4-5XSubMax

Neutral Grip Pull Ups> 4-5XSubMax

incline Bench DB Curls> 4-5X12

Finisher- Burpees 5X10 30-60sec rest between sets.

WOD 11

Sandbag Clean & Press X10

Pull Ups/Muscle Ups XSubMax

Alternating Jumping Split Squat X12ea

Pull Aparts X15

200M Run

25 Min AMRAP

WOD 12

Sandbag Squat X8-12

Bentover BB Row X10-15

Dips XSubMax

Jump Rope X100

AMRAP 15 mins

Box Jump X10

Push Ups w/ bands or chains XSubMax

Farmer Walks X100ft

Jump Rope X100

AMRAP 15 mins

WOD 13

Tire Flips 5X10

Mixed Grip Pull Ups 5XSubMax

KB Rack Front Squat 5X8

Snatch 5X12ea

Ab Roll Out 5X15

Tabata Rope Slams 1 cycle

WOD 14

400M Run

Speed Skater Split Squats X15ea

Rope Climb/Rope Pull ups X25ft/SubMax

Overhead Carry X100yds A5- Farmer Carry X100yd

400M Run

Repeat for 40 mins AMRAP

WOD 15

Bench Press 4X8

Single Arm DB Row 4X12-15

Incline DB Press 5X15

Inverted Row 5XSubMax

Bent Over Y Lateral Shoulder Raise 5X10
Finisher:

RKC Plank 20 sec followed by 10 burpees X5 rest
90 sec.

WOD 16

KB Front Squat X 15

Watercan Carry X 100M

Box Jump X 10

KB Swing X 20

Sandbag Carry X 200M

As many rounds as possible in 35 minutes.

WOD 17

Barbell Press X5-8

Pull Ups/Weighted XSubMax

Single Arm DB Clean n Press X10ea

Standing Barbell Twist X20

KB Swing X15

Finisher 1 Mile Loaded Carry

WOD 18

Sandbag Squat> 5X8

Sandbag Press> 5X10

Sledgehammer Slam> 5X45 Seconds

Farmer Walks> 5X100ft

Tire Flips> 5X10

WOD 19

Pull Ups 5XSubMax

Dips 5XSubMax

Burpee 5X5

Push Ups 5XSubMax

Inverted Row 5XSubMax

Wall Walk 5X5

Burpee 5X5

WOD 20

200 Push Ups

200 Air Squats

100 Inverted Rows

200 Lunges

200 Sit Ups

8 400M sprints

For time! You can break them up any way you want the goal is to complete it as fast as possible.

WOD 21

Bear Crawl X50/100 Meters

Rope Climb/Inverted Row X25ft(or equal to)/SubMax

Burpee 2 Push Ups X2 (5 burpees 10/20 push ups)

Sandbag/DB Shoulder 2 Shoulder Press X20 each side

Repeat 5 times

3 Mile Ruck Run For Time

WOD 22

SquatX50 with barbell or sandbag

400M Run

Pull Ups/Muslce UpsX25

400M Run

Clean&PressX15

800M Run

WOD 23

Fireman Carry> 5X100yds

Buddy Wheel Barrel> 5X50yds

Partner Battling Ropes> 5X30secs

Med Ball Squats 2 Buddy Toss> 5X30Sec

Partner Bear Crawls> 5X50yds

Jerry Can/Ammo Box Medley> 3X as fast as possible for time

Set up 5 sets of Jerry Cans full of water and 1 Ammo crate full of sand/dirty. One person will carry all 5 sets of jerry cans and the ammo crate for 30 yds, then the partner will carry each back for time with a total of 3 rounds.

WOD 24

Pull Ups> XSubMax

Step Ups> X15ea

Walking Lunges

Dips

Inverted Rows

Push Ups

Sprint 100M 40 min AMRAP for added difficulty wear a kit/weighted vets

WOD 25

Pull Ups> XSubMax

Step Ups> X15ea

Walking Lunges

Dips

Inverted Rows

Push Ups

Sprint 100M 40 min AMRAP for added difficutly wear a kit/weighted vets

WOD 26

Turkish Getups> x5 ea side

Spider Man Pushups> XSubMax

Walking Lunges> X20ea

Farmer Walk> X100M

400M Run

40 Min AMRAP

WOD 27

Tire Flips> X5-10

Pull Ups/Muslce Ups> XSubMax

Sandbag Shoulder Squat> X10ea (hold the sandbag on one shoulder for each set)

Wall Walks> X5-8

30mins as many rounds as possible

Finisher> Prowler/Sled SuicicdesX5

WOD 28

Deadlift> Work up to a 5RM

Pull Ups> 5XSubMax

Tire Flip> 3X5

Wheel Barrel Handwalks> 3X50ft

Walking Barbell Lunges> 4X10ea

Farmer Walks> 4x100ft

Finisher: Rower 30sec on 30 sec rest for 6 rounds

WOD 29

Sandbag Squat X15

Sandbag Shoulder to Shoulder Press X12

Rope Climb/Sled Rope Pull X UpDown/50ft

Heavy Sled Sprint X40yds

RowX 400M

Repeat for 5-6 Rounds for time.

WOD 30

Pull UpsX SubMax (These you can do on anything from an overhand to a tree)

Jump Squat X20

Wall Walk XSubMax   (Just find a wall and get to it)

Dips XSubMax (You can do these on a bench or the end of your trunk increase difficulty to single leg or legs elevated if needed)

Car Push X50ft (Get behind and push)

Perform for 5-10 rounds depending on your level of training and time in your trip.

WOD 31

Turkish Get Ups X5 each side

Pull Ups (bodyweight or with chains) XSubMax

Alternating Reverse Lunges w/ odd object X15 per leg

Clap Push Ups XSubMax

Sledge Hammer Slam X20

Jump Rope X100/50double unders

Repeat 5-6 rounds for time

After you will perform explosive jumps in the pool 5X3 then 15 mins of moderate intensity swimming 60-70%. If you do not have a pool you will perform weighted jump squats with 10lb dbs and row for 15mins at the same intensity.

WOD 32

50 pull ups. (Not Kipping)

50 burpees

50 lunges with 75 pound

1 mile ruck with 75 pound log

WOD 33

Jungle Gym Suspended Crunch 40

Tire Flips 10 (450/200)

Jungle Gym Pike Press 40

Sledge Slams 20/20 (20 on right, 20 on left)

Four Rounds For Time

WOD 34

Ruck 1 mile

50 lunges

40 burpees

30 lunges

20 burpees

10 lunges

10 burpees

Ruck 1 mile

WOD 35

Box JumpX5/10

Sledge Hammer Swings/Ball SlamX 15

Single Arm Overhead CarryX100ft

V-UpX20

Clap Push Ups into SprintXSubMax-200M

WOD 36

Front Squat

Double Jerk

Reverse Lunge

Double Clean

Front Lunge

Double Clean & Jerk

Thruster

Alternating Double Jerk

Reverse Lunge

Alternating Double Cleans

Front Lunge

Double Clean & Jerk

WOD 37

21 Thrusters (2 – 1.5 pood KBs), 12 ascents 15′ rope

21 Thrusters (2 – 1.5 pood KBs) 9 ascents 15′ rope

15 Thrusters (2 – 1.5 pood KBs) 6 ascents 15′ rope

WOD 38

10 Minutes:

5 Minutes KB Snatch Right (16 kg)

5 Minutes KB Snatch Left (16 kg)

Note: Try to maintain 16-20 reps per minute. Watch the clock, pace yourself, be efficient and "rest" on top.

Take a 5-10 minute break then...

Finish with 3 rounds of:

1 minute – 1 arm swings Left (24 kg)

1 minute – 1 arm swings Right (24 kg)

WOD 39

10 Minutes

As Many Reps As Possible:

TGU's – 24 kg KB

Alternate sides after each rep. Use strict form.
 Do not sacrifice form for reps !

Finish

5 – 50 yd Hill Sprints

WOD 40

5 rounds of 5

Performed in a circuit, 3 minute rest in between rounds

Deadlift (80% of 1 rep max)

Military Press (80% of 1 rep max) KB or BB

Weighted Pull-ups (80% of 1 rep max)

5 rounds

50 1-Arm KB Swings (alternating hands each rep)

10 Burpees

1 minute rest in between rounds

WOD 41

Warm-up

5 minutes SHOT Drills

Practice **5** H2H Drills - 1 round of each drill of choice;

2 Minute Rounds/ 30 seconds rest between rounds

WOD 42

21-15-9 for Time:

1 Arm Thruster R (24 kg)

1 Arm Thruster L (24 kg)

Pull-ups

WOD 43

Warm -up

5 Minutes H2H KB Drills (12 or 16 kg)

5 Rounds For time:

3 Deadlifts (90% of 1 rep max)

3 Pull-ups (32 kg)

3 Handstand Push-ups (Rings or parralettes)

Finish:

5 50 yard Sprints

WOD 44

5 rounds of the following:

3 Clean Pulls

3 Power Cleans

3 Push Press

3 Push Jerks

3 Good Mornings

*Perform at 60%-70% of 3 RM Power Clean

*Rest 2 minutes between rounds

WOD 45

5 rounds for time:

Sprint 100 yards

12 Snatches R/L – 24 kg KB

12 Pull Ups

WOD 46

10,9,8,7,6,5,4,3,2,1, for Time:

KB Thrusters (2 – 24 kg KBs)

Muscle-Ups

WOD 47

5 Rounds (90% 1 rep max)

3 Deadlifts

3 Weighted Pull-ups

3 Hand Stand Push-ups(parallettes)

5 Knees to Elbows

WOD 48

3 Rounds

10 Turkish Get-ups R/L (24 kg)

10 Muscle-Ups

WOD 49

4 Rounds for Time:

25 ring push ups

25 pull-ups

25 Swings (1.5 pood)

200m run

WOD 50

21 Thrusters (2 – 1.5 pood KBs), 12 ascents 15′ rope

21 Thrusters (2 – 1.5 pood KBs) 9 ascents 15′ rope

15 Thrusters (2 – 1.5 pood KBs) 6 ascents 15′ rope

WOD 51

Warm up

Joint Mobility Drills

AMRAP in 10 minutes

5 KB Snatch R/L (24 kg)

10 Wall Ball

5 Weighted Pull-ups (24 kg)

WOD 52

3 Rounds

10 Turkish Get-ups R/L (24 kg)

10 Muscle-Ups

WOD 53

Long Cycle + Pull-ups

10,9,8,7,6,5,4,3,2,1 reps for time

Double KB Clean & Jerk (24 kg men, 12 kg women)

Strict Pull ups (16 kg men, body weight women)

WOD 54

10,9,8,7,6,5,4,3,2,1 For Time:

KB Swing (32kg)

Ring Dips

Box Jumps

WOD 55

Tabada Format (20 seconds work 10 seconds rest)

8 rounds (12 minutes total)

KB Swings (24 kg)

Ring Push ups

Knees-to-Elbows

WOD 56

10 Reps Towards KB Perfection

For Time:

Prescribed weight – whatever you need to perform perfect reps. Perform 10 reps each arm for all one-arm exercises.

10 One-arm Floor Presses R/L

10 Arm-Bar Stretches R/L

10 Double Floor Presses

10 Turkish Get Ups R/L

10 Military Press R/L

10 Push-Presses R/L

10 Russian Swings

10 Power Swings

10 American Swings

10 Swing Releases

10 One-Arm Swings R/L

10 Half Rotations Switches

10 H2H Switches

10 KB Dead Cleans R/L

10 KB (Swing) Cleans R/L

10 Bottoms-up Cleans R/L

10 Double KB Cleans

10 Thrusters

10 Snatches R/L

WOD 56

5 Minutes of each drill:

SHOT Drills (8-12# shot)

H2H Drills (12-16 kg KB)

100 KB Snatch for time – alternate L/R as needed (24 kg/16kg)

WOD 57

5 Rounds for Time:

10 Thick Bar Hang Power Cleans (135#)

10 Double KB Military Presses (24 kg)

10 Pull-ups

WOD 58

15 Power Clean & Jerk (155#)

5 Handstand Push-ups

10 Power C & J (155#)

10 Handstand Push-ups

5 Power C & J (155#)

15 Handstand Push ups

WOD 59

AMRAP (as many rounds as possible) for 10 minutes (24 kg/16)

1 One-Arm Swing (r)

1 KB Clean (r)

1 KB Front Squat (r)

1 MP (r)

1 KB Snatch (r)

Repeat the sequence above with the left to finish Round 1.

Switch back to right hand and begin round 2... repeat for 10 minutes.

WOD 60

5 Rounds for time:

3 Power Cleans (165#)

3 Front Squats (165#)

1 Push Jerk (165#)

Note: Be very technical on the above lifts. Scale up or down as necessary.

Finish with 3 Rounds of:

3 Clean Grip High-Pulls (205#)

Note: The CGHPs are for power development, don't let a weak or taxed grip be the limiting factor on this lift, use straps, if necessary.5 Rounds for time:

WOD 61

Warm Up

500m row

5 Turkish Get-ups R/L (12 or 16 kg)

25 Snatches R/L (12 or 16 kg)

Tactical Athlete Total

Three attempts each at:

Back Squat

Double KB Military Press (start in the rack position, hand must be below chin, press to lockout)

Deadlift

Weighted Pull-up

WOD 62

Warm-up

100 One-Arm Swings (alternate L/R as needed) 16 kg

5 Rounds for Time:

5 Turkish Get-ups (R+L=1 rep) Alternate sides every rep – 24 kg

5 Muscle ups

WOD 63

Warm-up

500 meter row

50 One-Arm Swings (switch hands every rep)

30 Reps: for time:

Turkish Get-ups R/L =1 (16 or 24 kg)

Muscle ups

WOD 64

10 Reps Towards KB Perfection

For Time:

Prescribed weight – whatever you need to perform perfect reps. Perform 10 reps each arm for all one-arm exercises.

10 One-arm Floor Presses R/L

10 Arm-Bar Stretches R/L

10 Double Floor Presses

10 Turkish Get Ups R/L

10 Military Press R/L

10 Push-Presses R/L

10 Russian Swings

10 Power Swings

10 American Swings

10 Swing Releases

10 One-Arm Swings R/L

10 Half Rotations Switches

10 H2H Switches

10 KB Dead Cleans R/L

10 KB (Swing) Cleans R/L

10 Bottoms-up Cleans R/L

10 Double KB Cleans

10 Thrusters

10 Snatches R/L

WOD 65

10,9,8,7,6,5,4,3,2,1 reps for time

1.5 x BW Deadlift

1 x BW Bench Press* (or Double Kettlebells
Floor Press 2 – 40 kg KB)

.75 x BW Cleans

WOD 66

Joint Mobility Drills

AMRAP in 10 minutes

5 KB Snatch R/L (24 kg/16kg)

10 Wall Ball

5 Weighted Pull-ups (24 kg/16kg)

WOD 67

1000m row

50 KB Snatches R/L (16kg or 12 kg)

5×5 80% of 1 rep Max

Back Squat

Weighted Ring Dips

Janda Sit-ups

Weighted Chins

5 50 yd sprints

WOD 68

10,9,8,7,6,5,4,3,2,1 reps for time

1.5 x BW Deadlift

1 x BW Bench Press* (or Double Kettlebells
Floor Press 2 – 40 kg KB)

.75 x BW Cleans

WOD 69

10,9,8,7,6,5,4,3,2,1

KB Swing (32kg/24kg) Two-Hand Swing of
choice (i.e. Russian, American, 2-Hand Release)

Box Jumps

WOD 70

KB Snatches 50 reps per arm (Skill work: 12 – 16 kg)

H2H Kettlebell Drills (12 -16 kg) 5 minutes

Helen

3 rounds for time:

400m Run

21 American Swing (24 kg)

12 Pull-ups

WOD 71

Warm up

Row 1000 m

5 rounds for time:

5 Power Cleans 185 lbs

20 Double Unders

WOD 72

Warm up

5 minutes of H2H Kettlebell Drills (Keep it light and happy!)

AMRAP in 20 mins

2 Muscle ups

4 Handstand Pushups

8 KB Swings (32kg/24kg)

WOD 73

Warm up

500 m row

3 minutes SHOT Drills

5 rounds of 5

Performed in a circuit, 3 minute rest in between rounds

Squat (40-50% of 1 rep max)

Deadlift (80% of 1 rep max)

Military Press (80% of 1 rep max) KB or BB

Weighted Pull-ups (80% of 1 rep max)

Note: The purpose of performing a light weight low bar back squat is assist the dead lift. It will greatly enhance your ability to maintain an open chest – straight back at the starting position and for the duration of the pull.

WOD 74

5 Rounds for time:

3 Power Cleans (165#)

3 Front Squats (165#)

1 Push Jerk (165#)

Note: Be very technical on the above lifts. Scale up or down as necessary.

Finish with 3 Rounds of:

3 Clean Grip High-Pulls (205#)

Note: The CGHPs are for power development, don't let a weak or taxed grip be the limiting factor on this lift, use straps, if necessary.

WOD 75

Warm up

Joint Mobility Drills

AMRAP in 10 minutes

10 KB Snatch R/L (24 kg/16kg)

10 Wall Ball

5 Weighted Pull-ups (24 kg/16kg)

WOD 76

15-12-9 for Time:

Double KB Clean & Jerk (24 kg/16kg)

Ring Dips

Pull-ups

WOD 77

Warm-up

50 KB Snatches R/L (16 kg)

10 Knees to Elbows

3,3,3,3,3,3 85% of 1 Rep Max

Back Squat

Double KB Military Press (start in the rack position, hand must be below chin, press to lockout)

Deadlift

Weighted Pull-up

WOD 78

For Time:

15 Power Clean & Jerk (155#)

5 Handstand Push-ups

10 Power C & J (155#)

10 Handstand Push-ups

5 Power C & J (155#)

15 Handstand Push ups

WOD 79

10 Reps Towards KB Perfection

For Time:

Prescribed weight – whatever you need to perform perfect reps. Perform 10 reps each arm for all one-arm exercises.

10 One-arm Floor Presses R/L

10 Arm-Bar Stretches R/L

10 Double Floor Presses

10 Turkish Get Ups R/L

10 Military Press R/L

10 Push-Presses R/L

10 Russian Swings

10 Power Swings

10 American Swings

10 Swing Releases

10 One-Arm Swings R/L

10 Half Rotations Switches

10 H2H Switches

10 KB Dead Cleans R/L

10 KB (Swing) Cleans R/L

10 Bottoms-up Cleans R/L

10 Double KB Cleans

10 Thrusters

10 Snatches R/L

WOD 80

5 Rounds for time:

1000 Meter Row

5 KB Snatches R/L (32 kg)

WOD 81

10,9,8,7,6,5,4,3,2,1

KB Swing (32kg/24kg) = Two Hand Swing of choice (i.e. Russian, American, Swing Release)

Box Jumps

WOD 82

Kettlebell Fran

21-15-9 for time:

Double KB Clean & Jerk (2 – 16 kg men/ 12 kg women)

Pull-up

WOD 83

AMRAP in 20 Minutes

3 Muscle-ups

5 KB Swings (24 kg)

7 Box Jumps

WOD 84

As many rounds as possible in 12 minutes:

3 Handstand Push Ups

5 Pull Ups

7 Knees to Elbows

Cool Down:

2 minutes Pummeling Drill with partner or Shadow Box

WOD 85

Tabada Format (20 seconds work 10 seconds rest)

8 rounds (12 minutes total)

KB Swings (24 kg)

Ring Push ups

Knees-to-Elbows

WOD 86

10 Reps Towards KB Perfection

For Time:

Prescribed weight – whatever you need to perform perfect reps. Perform 10 reps each arm for all one-arm exercises.

10 One-arm Floor Presses R/L

10 Arm-Bar Stretches R/L

10 Double Floor Presses

10 Turkish Get Ups R/L

10 Military Press R/L

10 Push-Presses R/L

10 Russian Swings

10 Power Swings

10 American Swings

10 Swing Releases

10 One-Arm Swings R/L

10 Half Rotations Switches

10 H2H Switches

10 KB Dead Cleans R/L

10 KB (Swing) Cleans R/L

10 Bottoms-up Cleans R/L

10 Double KB Cleans

10 Thrusters

10 Snatches R/L

WOD 87

5 Minutes of each drill:

SHOT Drills (8-12# shot)

H2H Drills (12-16 kg KB)

100 KB Snatch for time – alternate L/R as needed (24 kg)

WOD 88

5 Rounds for Time:

10 Thick Bar Hang Power Cleans (135#)

10 Double KB Military Presses (24 kg)

10 Pull-ups

WOD 89

15 Power Clean & Jerk (155#)

5 Handstand Push-ups

10 Power C & J (155#)

10 Handstand Push-ups

5 Power C & J (155#)

15 Handstand Push ups

WOD 90

10 rounds for time (24 kg)

1 One-Arm Swing (r)

1 KB Clean (r)

1 KB Front Squat (r)

1 MP (r)

1 KB Snatch (r)

Repeat the sequence above with the left to finish Round 1. Switch back to right hand and begin round 2... repeat for 10 rounds.

WOD 91

5 Rounds for time:

3 Power Cleans (165#)

3 Front Squats (165#)

1 Push Jerk (165#)

Note: Be very technical on the above lifts. Scale up or down as necessary.

Finish with 3 Rounds of:

3 Clean Grip High-Pulls (205#)

Note: The CGHPs are for power development, don't let a weak or taxed grip be the limiting factor on this lift, use straps, if necessary.5 Rounds for time:

WOD 92

500m row

5 Turkish Get-ups R/L (12 or 16 kg)

25 Snatches R/L (12 or 16 kg)

Tactical Athlete Total

Three attempts each at:

Back Squat

Double KB Military Press (start in the rack position, hand must be below chin, press to lockout)

Deadlift

Weighted Pull-up

The CrossFit Total was created by mark Rippetoe. He compiled the three most effective lifts for developing functional strength into one contest. Now, all you have to do is add the weighted pull-up. Be sure to pull with your palms facing out and make sure the front of your neck (not your chin) touches the bar; otherwise it's just a good try.

WOD 92

Warm-up

100 One-Arm Swings (alternate L/R as needed) 16 kg

5 Rounds for Time:

5 Turkish Get-ups (R+L=1 rep) Alternate sides every rep – 24 kg

5 Muscle ups

WOD 93

Warm-up

500 meter row

50 One-Arm Swings (switch hands every rep)

30 Reps: for time:

Turkish Get-ups R/L =1 (16 or 24 kg)

Muscle ups

WOD 94

10 Reps Towards KB Perfection

For Time:

Prescribed weight – whatever you need to perform perfect reps. Perform 10 reps each arm for all one-arm exercises.

10 One-arm Floor Presses R/L

10 Arm-Bar Stretches R/L

10 Double Floor Presses

10 Turkish Get Ups R/L

10 Military Press R/L

10 Push-Presses R/L

10 Russian Swings

10 Power Swings

10 American Swings

10 Swing Releases

10 One-Arm Swings R/L

10 Half Rotations Switches

10 H2H Switches

10 KB Dead Cleans R/L

10 KB (Swing) Cleans R/L

10 Bottoms-up Cleans R/L

10 Double KB Cleans

10 Thrusters

10 Snatches R/L

WOD 95

Linda (KB)

10,9,8,7,6,5,4,3,2,1 reps for time

1.5 x BW Deadlift

1 x BW Bench Press* (or Double Kettlebells
Floor Press 2 – 40 kg KB)

.75 x BW Cleans

WOD 96

Warm up

Joint Mobility Drills

AMRAP in 10 minutes

5 KB Snatch R/L (24 kg)

10 Wall Ball

5 Weighted Pull-ups (24 kg)

WOD 97

Warm-up

1000m row

50 KB Snatches R/L (16kg or 12 kg)

WOD

5×5 80% of 1 rep Max

Back Squat

Weighted Ring Dips

Janda Sit-ups

Weighted Chins

Finish

5 50 yd sprints

WOD 98

10,9,8,7,6,5,4,3,2,1 reps for time

1.5 x BW Deadlift

1 x BW Bench Press* (or Double Kettlebells
Floor Press 2 – 40 kg KB)

.75 x BW Cleans

WOD 99

10,9,8,7,6,5,4,3,2,1

KB Swing (32kg)

Box Jumps

WOD 100

Warm-Up

KB Snatches 50 reps per arm (Skill work: 12 – 16 kg)

H2H Kettlebell Drills (12 -16 kg) 5 minutes

Helen

3 rounds for time:

400m Run

21 American Swing (24 kg)

12 Pull-ups

WOD 101

Warm up

Row 1000 m

5 rounds for time:

5 Power Cleans 185 lbs

20 Double Unders

WOD 102

Warm up

5 minutes of H2H Kettlebell Drills (Keep it light and happy!)

AMRAP in 20 mins

2 Muscle ups

4 Handstand Pushups

8 KB Swings (2 pood)

WOD 103

Warm up

500 m row

3 minutes SHOT Drills

5 rounds of 5

Performed in a circuit, 3 minute rest in between rounds

Squat (40-50% of 1 rep max)

Deadlift (80% of 1 rep max)

Military Press (80% of 1 rep max) KB or BB

Weighted Pull-ups (80% of 1 rep max)

Note: The purpose of performing a light weight low bar back squat is assist the dead lift. It will greatly enhance your ability to maintain an open chest – straight back at the starting position and for the duration of the pull.

WOD 104

5 Rounds for time:

3 Power Cleans (165#)

3 Front Squats (165#)

1 Push Jerk (165#)

Note: Be very technical on the above lifts. Scale up or down as necessary.

Finish with 3 Rounds of:

3 Clean Grip High-Pulls (205#)

Note: The CGHPs are for power development, don't let a weak or taxed grip be the limiting factor on this lift, use straps, if necessary.

WOD 105

Warm up

Joint Mobility Drills

AMRAP in 10 minutes

5 KB Snatch R/L (24 kg)

10 Wall Ball

5 Weighted Pull-ups (24 kg)

WOD 106

15-12-9 for Time:

Double KB Clean & Jerk (24 kg)

Ring Dips

Pull-ups

WOD 107

Warm-up

50 KB Snatches R/L (16 kg)

10 Knees to Elbows

3,3,3,3,3,3 85% of 1 Rep Max

Back Squat

Double KB Military Press (start in the rack position, hand must be below chin, press to lockout)

Deadlift

Weighted Pull-up

WOD 108

For Time:

15 Power Clean & Jerk (155#)

5 Handstand Push-ups

10 Power C & J (155#)

10 Handstand Push-ups

5 Power C & J (155#)

15 Handstand Push ups

WOD 109

10 Reps Towards KB Perfection

For Time:

Prescribed weight – whatever you need to perform perfect reps. Perform 10 reps each arm for all one-arm exercises.

10 One-arm Floor Presses R/L

10 Arm-Bar Stretches R/L

10 Double Floor Presses

10 Turkish Get Ups R/L

10 Military Press R/L

10 Push-Presses R/L

10 Russian Swings

10 Power Swings

10 American Swings

10 Swing Releases

10 One-Arm Swings R/L

10 Half Rotations Switches

10 H2H Switches

10 KB Dead Cleans R/L

10 KB (Swing) Cleans R/L

10 Bottoms-up Cleans R/L

10 Double KB Cleans

10 Thrusters

10 Snatches R/L

WOD 110

5 Rounds for time:

1000 Meter Row

5 KB Snatches R/L (32 kg)

WOD 111

21-15-9 for time:

Double KB Clean & Jerk (2 – 24 kg)

Muscle-Up

WOD 112

10 Reps Towards KB Perfection

For Time:

Prescribed weight – whatever you need to perform perfect reps. Perform 10 reps each arm for all one-arm exercises.

10 One-arm Floor Presses R/L

10 Arm-Bar Stretches R/L

10 Double Floor Presses

10 Turkish Get Ups R/L

10 Military Press R/L

10 Push-Presses R/L

10 Russian Swings

10 Power Swings

10 American Swings

10 Swing Releases

10 One-Arm Swings R/L

10 Half Rotations Switches

10 H2H Switches

10 KB Dead Cleans R/L

10 KB (Swing) Cleans R/L

10 Bottoms-up Cleans R/L

10 Double KB Cleans

10 Thrusters

10 Snatches R/L

WOD 113

5 Rounds for time:

5 Power Cleans (85% of 1 rep max)

5 Muscle ups

5 Handstand Push-ups

WOD 114

Strength

Weighted Pull-ups 4 x Max Effort @ Heaviest possible

*you should be able to perform at least 3 reps if not more with the weight you choose, if you cannot complete 3 lighten the load

Conditioning

6 Rounds For Time Of:

30 ft. Low Crawl

20 x Sit-Ups

10 x Squats w/ 40lb. Sandbag

200m Run w/ 40lb. Sandbag

5 x Strict Pull-Ups

Water Work

-6 x 100m Intervals (freestyle), as fast as possible, rest 1:1

*6 sets of 100 meter swim sprints in the stroke of your choice, each interval should be full speed, rest is equal to the amount of time it took for the 100m interval.

-Drown proofing practice (10-15 minutes of total practice)(for this exercise, without using hands or feet, exhale and sink to the bottom of the pool, jump off the bottom of the pool to come back up for air, take a breath and repeat)

*DO NOT complete the underwater or breath holding practice alone, these should be done in guarded waters and with a swim buddy NO EXCEPTIONS.

WOD 115

Strength

Back Squat 2 x 15 @ 65% (high bar only)

*weight should be 65% of your 1 repetition max for 2 sets of 15 reps

Conditioning

For Time:

800m Run

20 x Strict Pull-ups

800m Run

40 x Push-ups

800m Run

10 x Strict Pull-ups

800m Run

20 x Push-ups

Water Work

-12 x 25m Intervals (freestyle), as fast as possible, rest 2:1

*12 sets of 25 meter swim sprints in the stroke of your choice, each interval should be full speed, rest is double the amount of time it took for the 25m interval.

-25m Underwater Swim Practice (15-20 Minutes, take adequate rest between attempts)

*DO NOT complete the underwater or breath holding practice alone, these should be done in guarded waters and

WOD 116

<u>Strength</u>

Bench Press 3 x 15 @ Heaviest Possible

*weight should be heaviest possible for 15 reps but you must complete all 15 reps of each set without failure. For every rep failed perform 10 Burpees

Conditioning

5 Rounds For Time:

20 x Split Jumps (jump lunges)

60 ft. Bear Crawl

10 x Burpee + 3 Push-ups

60 ft. Bear Crawl

10 x Strict Pull-ups

*for Burpee + 3 Push-ups perform a standard burpee and when in the bottom position complete 3 full range of motion push-ups before finishing the burpee.

Water Work

-8 x 50m Intervals (freestyle), as fast as possible, rest 2:1

*8 sets of 50 meter swim sprints in the stroke of your choice, each interval should be full speed, rest is double the amount of time it took for the 50m interval.

-25m Underwater Swim Practice (15-20 Minutes, take adequate rest between attempts)

*DO NOT complete the underwater or breath holding practice alone, these should be done in guarded waters and with a swim buddy, NO EXCEPTIONS

WOD 117

Sit-Up Test – After warming up perform 2 minutes of UNBROKEN Sit-UPS, as many as possible (this is your baseline sit-up number, once the clock starts rest is allowed, only in the up position with elbows touching within 3 inches) of the knees

*hands must always be in contact with your opposite shoulders, full range of motion is shoulder blades must contact the ground at bottom and elbows must touch 3 inches below the knees at a minimum

Conditioning

2 Rounds for time of:

50 x flutter kicks (3 count)

40 x Burpees

30 x Push-ups

20 x Pull-ups

100 meter Sprint

<u>Water Work</u>

For Time:

1000m swim (combat side stroke only)
*if you do not have the combat side stroke down well enough to swim 1000m, practice technique for 30 minutes

WOD 118

1.5 Mile test – After warming up perform a max effort 1.5 Mile run for time (even if your PFT requires a 2 Mile run perform this 1.5 Mile test)

*post times to comments

Conditioning

6 Rounds

5 x Strict Pull-ups

10 x Push-ups

15 x Sit-ups

20 x Squats

Water Work

-10 x 25m Intervals (freestyle), as fast as possible, rest 2:1

*10 sets of 25 meter swim sprints in the stroke of your choice, each interval should be full speed, rest is double the amount of time it took for the 25m interval.

-Drown proofing practice (10-15 minutes of total practice)(for this exercise, without using hands or feet, exhale and sink to the bottom of the pool, jump off the bottom of the pool to come back up for air, take a breath and repeat)

*DO NOT complete the underwater or breath holding practice alone, these should be done in guarded waters and with a swim buddy, NO EXCEPTIONS

WOD 119

Push-Up Test — After warming up perform 2 minutes of UNBROKEN PUSH-UPS, as many as possible (this is your baseline push-up number, once the clock starts no rest is allowed)

*elbows must be fully locked out at the top and chest must be at least 3 inches from the ground at the bottom, have a friend keep there fist below your chest or use a sponge/block

Conditioning

400m Run

Max Effort Unbroken Pull-Ups

Rest 1:1

400m Run

Max Effort Unbroken Sit-Ups

Rest 1:1

400m Run

Max Effort Unbroken Push-Ups

Rest 1:1

400m Run

Max Effort Unbroken Sit-Ups

*Max Effort means you are performing as many reps of the given exercise as possible without rest, the set is over when you break or fail.

*Your rest is equal to the amount of time it takes you to complete the 400m run to the last rep before failure of the exercise you are on

Water Work

-5 x 100m Intervals (freestyle), as fast as possible, rest 1:1

*5 sets of 100 meter swim sprints in the stroke of your choice, each interval should be full speed,

rest is equal to the amount of time it took for the 100m interval.

-25 meter underwater swim practice (10-15 minutes of total practice time)

*DO NOT complete the underwater or breath holding practice alone, these should be done in guarded waters and with a swim buddy, NO EXCEPTIONS.

WOD 120

Pull-Up Test – After warming up perform 1 set of STRICT, UNBROKEN PULL-UPS, as many as possible (this is your baseline pull-up number)

*chin must clearly pass over the top of the bar and you must be fully extended at the bottom of each rep in the hang position

Conditioning

6 Rounds for Time of:

10 x Burpees

200m Run

20 x Body Squats

200m Run

Water Work

-8 x 50m Intervals (freestyle), as fast as possible, rest 1:1

*8 sets of 50 meter swim sprints in the stroke of your choice, each interval should be full speed, rest is equal to the amount of time it took for the 50m interval.

-25 meter underwater swim practice (10-15 minutes of total practice time)

*DO NOT complete the underwater or breath holding practice alone, these should be done in guarded waters and with a swim buddy, NO EXCEPTIONS.

WOD 121

5 Rounds of:

20 x Push-ups

20 x Sit-ups

200m Run

*1 Minute Rest between rounds

WATER WORK

For Time:

500m Swim, combat side stroke or breast stroke only

*This swim is to determine a baseline of where you stand at the beginning of this programming. If you are unable to perform 1 of these 2 strokes spend 15-20 minutes practicing the combat side stroke.

WOD 122

Strength

Bench Press 4 x 12 @ Heaviest Possible

*weight should be heaviest possible for 12 reps but you must complete all 12 reps of each set without failure. For every rep failed perform 10 Burpees

Conditioning

Run 3 Miles then:

Pyramid of pull-ups and push-ups

1 up to 10 then back down

Double the number of push-ups

(1 pull-up / 2 push-ups, 2 pull-ups / 4 push-ups, ect.)

Water Work

-8 x 100m Intervals (Combat Side Stroke/ Breast Stroke), as fast as possible, rest 2:00 minutes

*8 sets of 100 meter swims, each interval should be full speed, rest is 2:00 minutes.

-25m Underwater Swim Practice (15-20 Minutes, take adequate rest between attempts)

WOD 123

Strength

Back Squat 4 x 10 @ Heaviest Possible

*weight should be heaviest possible for 10 reps but you must complete all 10 reps of each set without failure. For every rep failed perform 10 Burpees

Conditioning

For Time:

500m Swim

20 x Push-ups

400m Swim

30 x Push-ups

300m Swim

40 x Push-ups

200m Swim

60 x Push-ups

100m Swim

*if a pool is unavailable, you may use a rower instead but must double each distance.

WOD 124

Strength

Bench Press 4 x 10 @ Heaviest Possible

*weight should be heaviest possible for 10 reps but you must complete all 10 reps of each set without failure. For every rep failed perform 10 Burpees

Conditioning

In an 8 hour time period (maximum) accumulate the following total reps and mileage (water work is included in conditioning):

Run 6 miles

300 x Push-ups

200 x sit-ups

100 x Pull-ups

Swim 2 miles

This should all be done In the shortest time period possible but if you must break it up due to time constraints make it happen in under 8 hours.

WOD 125

Strength

Shoulder Strict Press 4 x 12 @ Heaviest Possible

*weight should be heaviest possible for 12 reps but you must complete all 12 reps of each set without failure. For every rep failed perform 10 Burpees

Conditioning

For Time:

1.5 Mile Run

50 x Strict Pull-Ups

100 x Push-ups

100 x Sit-Ups

1.5 Mile Run

Water Work

-5 x 250m Intervals (Combat Side Stroke/ Breast Stroke), as fast as possible, rest 2:00 minutes

*5 sets of 250 meter swims, each interval should be full speed, rest is 2:00 minutes.

-25m Underwater Swim Practice (15-20 Minutes, take adequate rest between attempts)

WOD 126

Strength

Weighted Dips 4 x Max Effort @ Heaviest possible

*you should be able to perform at least 3 reps if not more with the weight you choose, if you cannot complete 3 lighten the load

Conditioning

5 Rounds for Max Reps:

-Push-ups

-Strict Pull-Ups

*Each round you will perform as many push-ups as possible until failure without rest, then perform as many strict pull-ups as possible without coming off the bar. No rest between rounds.

Water Work

- 10 x 50m Swim

*no fins, combat side stroke preferred

-Drown proofing practice (10-15 minutes of total practice)(for this exercise, without using hands or feet, exhale and sink to the bottom of the pool, jump off the bottom of the pool to come back up for air, take a breath and repeat)

WOD 127

Strength

Weighted Pull-ups 4 x Max Effort @ Heaviest possible

*you should be able to perform at least 3 reps if not more with the weight you choose, if you cannot complete 3 lighten the load

Conditioning

3 Rounds For Time Of:

200m Run w/ Sandbag (40lbs.)

20 x Incline Push-Ups (feet on ~20″ box)

200m Run w/ Sandbag (40lbs.)

20 x weighted Sit-Ups (holding 20lbs., dumbell, kettlebell, ect.)

200m Run w/ Sandbag (40lbs.)

10 x Strict Pull-Ups

 Water Work)

-6 x 100m Intervals (freestyle), as fast as possible, rest 1:1

*6 sets of 100 meter swim sprints in the stroke of your choice, each interval should be full speed, rest is equal to the amount of time it took for the 100m interval.

-Drown proofing practice (10-15 minutes of total practice)(for this exercise, without using hands or feet, exhale and sink to the bottom of the pool, jump off the bottom of the pool to come back up for air, take a breath and repeat)

WOD 128

Strength

Bench Press 3 x 15 @ Heaviest Possible

*weight should be heaviest possible for 15 reps but you must complete all 15 reps of

each set without failure. For every rep failed perform 10 Burpees

Conditioning

800m Run

2:00 minutes Max Effort (ME) Push-Ups

800m Run

2:00 ME Sit-Ups

800m Run

2:00 ME Pull-Ups

800m Run

2:00 ME Push-Ups

800m Run

Water Work

-2 x 800m Intervals (Combat Side Stroke/ Breast Stroke), as fast as possible, rest 2:00 minutes

*2 sets of 800 meter swims, each interval should be full speed, rest is 2:00 minutes.

-25m Underwater Swim Practice (15-20 Minutes, take adequate rest between attempts)

WOD 129

Strength

Strict Press 3 x 12 @ heaviest possible

*Weight should be heavy but you should not fail before 12 repetitions

Conditioning

4 Rounds for time of:

400m Run

50 x flutter kicks (3 count)

5 x rope climb (15 ft. = 1)

*if a climbing rope is not available perform 15 strict pull ups per round instead

Water Work

-4 x 250m Intervals (combat side stroke or breast stroke only), rest 3:1

*10 sets of 25 meter intervals each interval should be full speed, rest is triple the the amount of time it took for the 25m interval.

-25m Underwater Swim Practice (15-20 Minutes, take adequate rest between attempts)

WOD 130

Strength

Strict Press 3 x 12 @ heaviest possible

*Weight should be heavy but you should not fail before 12 repetitions

Conditioning

4 Rounds for time of:

400m Run

50 x flutter kicks (3 count)

5 x rope climb (15 ft. = 1)

*if a climbing rope is not available perform 15 strict pull ups per round instead

Water Work

-4 x 250m Intervals (combat side stroke or breast stroke only), rest 3:1

*10 sets of 25 meter intervals each interval should be full speed, rest is triple the the amount of time it took for the 25m interval.

-25m Underwater Swim Practice (15-20 Minutes, take adequate rest between attempts)

WOD 131

Strength

Back Squat 2 x 15 @ 65% (high bar only)

*weight should be 65% of your 1 repetition max for 2 sets of 15 reps

Conditioning

For Time:

3 Mile Run

Water Work

-4 x 250m Intervals (combat side stroke or breast stroke only), rest 1:2

*4 sets of 250 meter swims each interval should be full speed, rest is half the amount of time it took for the 250m interval.

-25m Underwater Swim Practice (15-20 Minutes, take adequate rest between attempts)

WOD 132

Strength

Weighted Dips 4 x Max Effort @ Heaviest possible

*you should be able to perform at least 3 reps if not more with the weight you choose, if you cannot complete 3 lighten the load

Conditioning

For Time:

8 minute Max Effort Run (for distance)

100 x Push-ups

4 minute Max Effort Run (for distance)

100 x Sit-ups

2 minute Max Effort Run (for distance)

50 x Strict Pull-ups

Water Work

-1 mile swim (1600m) for time

*no fins, combat side stroke preferred

-Drown proofing practice (10-15 minutes of total practice)(for this exercise, without using hands or feet, exhale and sink to the bottom of the pool, jump off the bottom of the pool to come back up for air, take a breath and repeat)

WOD 133

Agility

18-15-12-9-6-3 Wall Balls

18-15-12-9-6-3 Burpees

18-15-12-9-6-3 Push-ups

18-15-12-9-6-3 T2B (toes 2 bar)

WOD 134

Endurance

4 rounds for time

10 tire flips

25 wall balls

50 kettlebell swings

100 rope waves

100m farmers carry

WOD 135

Agility

5 rounds for time

10 burpees

10 deadlifts

20 renegade rows

20 push-ups

3- sit-ups

20 medicine ball slams

WOD 136

AMRAP for 15 minutes

10 Kettlebell sit-ups

10 Kettlebell swings

10 Kettlebell squats

WOD 137

Endurance

EMOTM for 15 minutes

10 squats

10 push-ups

10 T2B (toes 2 bar)

10 burpees

10 pull-ups

WOD 138

Agility

AMRAP for 20 minutes

5 burpees

5 squats

5 T2B (toes 2 bar)

WOD 139

Endurance

5 Rounds for time

30 medicine ball push-ups

30 wall balls

30 medicine ball slams

30 medicine ball sit-ups

WOD 140

Strength

EMOTM for 20 minutes

8 military press

8 pull-ups

8 ground to overhead

WOD 141

Power

4 rounds for time

10 deadlifts

10 back squats

10 bench press

10 front squats

WOD 142

Power & Endurance

10 rounds for time

50 yard dumbbell farmers carry

5 ground to overheads

5 thrusters

5 hang cleans

WOD 143

Power

10 rounds for time

5 weighted pull-ups

15 thrusters

10 deadlifts

8 deadlifts

WOD 143

Power

3 rounds for time

20 TGU (Turkish get up)

20 Kettlebell swings

20 Military press

WOD 144

Endurance

5 rounds for time

400m run

4 weighted pull-ups

4 rope climbs

4 front squats

4 handstand push-ups

4 clean and jerks

4 thrusters

WOD 145

Power

7 rounds for time

3 deadlifts

3 thrusters

3 pull-ups

3 snatches

3 cleans

3 handstand push-ups

WOD 146

AMRAP in 25 minutes

10 Kettlebell pistol squats

10 handstand push-ups

10 burpee pull-ups

10 thrusters

WOD 147

Power

4 Rounds for time

400m run

20 Kettlebell swings

20 box jumps

20 Kettlebell squats

WOD 148

Endurance

2 rounds for time

50 deadlifts

50 push-ups

50 Kettlebell swings

50 T2B (toes 2 bar)

WOD 149

Power/Endurance

10 rounds for time

10 thrusters

10 burpees

10 push press

10 burpees

10 thrusters

10 push press

WOD 150

Power

AMRAP in 20 minutes

30 bench press

30 burpees

30 deadlifts

30 jumping squats

30 barbell lunges

Conclusion

I hope you enjoy the plethora of workouts the Tactical Cross Training WOD Bible has to offer you, by following these workouts on a regular basis you'll develop not only a strong, flexible, functionally fit body that'll be ready to tackle any situation life throws at it but also an unbreakable mindset and confidence to match.

Whether you're looking to defend your country, get a competitive advantage in your sport, become a superhuman or just want to increase your mobility, strength and health these workouts are the answer.

I hope you enjoyed reading this book as much as I enjoyed writing it.

Would You Do Me A Favor?

I'm positive that if you follow the advice and WODs contained in this book your strength, endurance and agility will reach an all-time high.

I have one small favor to ask – Would you mind taking a minute to write a blurb onb Amazon about this book? I love getting feedback from my readers and hearing all of the success stories from individuals who have transformed their lives after reading my books.

You can leave me a review by visiting the following URL:

www.bitly.com/wodbible-review

Also, if you have any friends or family that might enjoy this book, spread the wisdom and lend it to them!

Books By P Selter

Visit www.WodBible.com to learn more about these books!

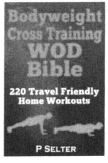 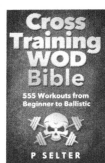 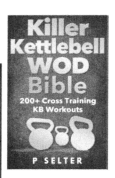

Bodyweight Cross Training WOD Bible: 220 Travel Friendly Home Workouts

Cross Training WOD Bible: 555 Workouts From Beginner to Ballistic

Killer Kettlebell WOD Bible: 200+ Cross Training KB Workouts

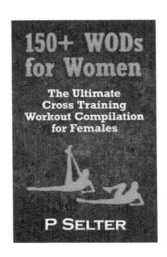

150+ WODs for Women: The Ultimate Cross Training Workout Compilation for Females

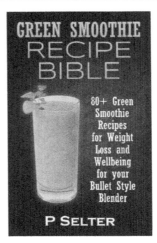

Green Smoothie Recipe Bible

Made in the USA
Monee, IL
04 December 2022

19653864R00069